50 Vegan Slow Cooker Recipes

Delicious Meatless Slow Cooker Meals For The Vegan Lifestyle

By Rachel Richards

© Revelry Publishing 2015

Copyright 2015 by Revelry Publishing

All Rights reserved under International and Pan-American Copyright Conventions. By payment of required fees, you have been granted the non-exclusive, non-transferable right to access and read the text of this book. No part of this text may be reproduced, transmitted, downloaded, decompiled, reverse-engineered or stored in or introduced into any information storage and retrieval system, in any form or by any means, whether electronic or mechanical, now known, hereinafter invented, without express written permission of the publisher.

DISCLAIMER

All information in this book has been carefully researched and checked for factual accuracy. However, the authors and publishers make no warranty, express or implied, that the information contained herein is appropriate for every individual, situation or purpose, and assume no responsibility for errors or omissions. The reader assumes the risk and full responsibility for all actions, and the authors will not be held responsible for any loss or damage, whether consequential, incidental, special or otherwise that may result from the information presented in this publication.

We have relied on our own experience as well as many different sources for this book, and we have done our best to check facts and to give credit where it is due. In the event that any material is incorrect or has been used without proper permission, please contact us so that the oversight can be corrected.

ISBN-13: 978-1987863291
ISBN-10: 1987863291

Other books by Rachel Richards:

The 7-Day Ketogenic Diet Meal Plan: 35 Delicious Low Carb Recipes For Weight Loss Motivation - Volume 1

The first volume of the set contains 35 different recipes and a bonus of a recipe for 'Keto Rolls'.

The 7-Day Ketogenic Diet Meal Plan: 35 Delicious Low Carb Recipes For Weight Loss Motivation - Volume 2

The second volume of the set contains 35 different recipes and a bonus of a recipe for 'Keto Almond Bread'.

The 7-Day Ketogenic Diet Meal Plan: 35 Delicious Low Carb Recipes For Weight Loss Motivation - Volume 3

The third volume of the set contains 35 different recipes and a bonus of a recipe for 'Posh Coffee'.

The 7-Day Ketogenic Diet Meal Plan: 35 Delicious Low Carb Recipes For Weight Loss Motivation - Volumes 1 to 3

This book has all three volumes of the set containing 105 different recipes and their respective bonuses of recipes for 'Keto Rolls', 'Keto Almond Bread' and 'Posh Coffee'.

The 7-Day Gluten Free Diet Plan: 35 Healthy Wheat Free Recipes To Banish Your Wheat Belly - Volume 1

This book was written for those who prefer food that is gluten-free whether it is for health reasons or simply a lifestyle choice.

Get the latest update on new releases from the author at:

https://rachelrichardsrecipebooks.com/newsletter

Table of Contents

Introduction 1
7 Day Vegan Meal Plan 2
7 Day Vegan Meal Plan Shopping List 4
Daily Fresh Purchases 6
Bonus 10
Breakfast 11
   1 - Cinnamon Apple Oatmeal 13
   2 - Vanilla Fig Oatmeal 15
   3 - Walnut Maple Pear Oatmeal 16
   4 - Carrot Cardamom Oatmeal 18
   5 - Strawberry Cake Oatmeal 19
   6 - Banana Pudding Oatmeal 20
   7 - Blueberry Coconut Quinoa 22
   8 - Breakfast Quinoa 23
   9 - Lemon Blueberry Muffin Oatmeal 24
   10 - Almond Milk Vanilla Spice Oatmeal 26
Soups and Stews 27
   11 - Ratatouille 28
   12 - Vegan Cassoulet 30
   13 - Spicy Black Bean Soup 31
   14 - Vegan Gumbo 32
   15 - Farro and Veggie Split Pea Soup 33
   16 - Vegan Greek Stew 35
   17 - Lentil Soup 36
   18 - Eggplant and Tomato Garbanzo Bean Stew 37
   19 - Vegan Pumpkin Chicken Chowder 38
   20 - Black Beans and Rice Soup 40
   21 - Black Bean-Chipotle Chili 41
   22 - Navy Bean Soup 42
   23 - Bean Stew 43
   24 - Black Bean Soup 45
   25 - Vegan Ethiopian Chicken Stew 47
   26 - Azorean Vegan Stew 48
   27 - Vegan Chicken and Sweet Potato Southwestern Stew 49

    28 - Vegan Cowboy Stew 51
    29 - Vegan Lamb Tagine 52
    30 - Vegan Sausage and Bean Stew 53
Main Dishes 54
    31 - Saag Aloo 55
    32 - Vegan "Soda Pop" Meatballs 57
    33 - Vegetable and Chickpea Curry 58
    34 - Homemade Applesauce 60
    35 - Lentil Bolognese 61
    36 - Vegetable Curry with Sweet Potato & Chickpeas .. 63
    37 - Butternut Squash 65
    38 - Tangy Vegan Meatballs 66
    39 - Chipotle Style Black Beans 67
    40 - Vegan Chili 68
Desserts 70
    41 - Poached Pears In Caramel Sauce 71
    42 - Peanut Butter Chocolate Slow Cooker Cake 73
    43 - Creamsicle Tapioca Pudding 75
    44 - Rice Pudding 77
    45 - Healthy Brownies 78
    46 - Apple Cobbler 80
    47 - Pumpkin Pie Pudding 81
    48 - Pumpkin Bread 82
    49 - Banana Brown Betty 84
    50 - Vegan Fudge 85
Thank You 87
Other Books by Rachel Richards 88
About the Author – Rachel Richards 89
Connect with Rachel Richards 90

For The Vegan Lifestyle

Introduction

What you eat has been proven to directly link to how you feel, function, and live. Everyone has heard the saying "you are what you eat," but not everyone realizes how true it really is. Essentially, if you fill your body with junk, you are going to feel like junk.

Once you begin to explore healthier options of what should be eaten, the findings are overwhelming: organic, non-GMO, fat-free, zero calories, low carbohydrates, high protein. The obsession of what to eat and what not to eat has become a constant battle for many. The solution is quite simple: vegan living.

A vegan's source of food can only come from non-animal products, including their meat, eggs, dairy, etc. The diet consists of mostly fruit, vegetables, wheat, rice, and legumes. The reasons for eating a vegan diet may vary, but many are health related. Going vegan will make you feel healthier, look better, and feel new.

A drawback to a vegan lifestyle is finding food. A vast majority of today's meals are not vegan friendly. The best way to insure that a meal is truly vegan is to prepare it at home, but the task does not even require more than ten minutes of time! A slow cooker is an efficient and delicious way to prepare vegan meals. Just add ingredients, let sit for a few hours, and then serve.

7 Day Vegan Meal Plan

Day One:

Breakfast - Banana Pudding Oatmeal
Lunch - Azorean Vegan Stew
Dinner - Ratatouille
Dessert - Banana Brown Betty

Day Two:

Breakfast - Walnut Maple Pear Oatmeal
Lunch - Vegan Cowboy Stew
Dinner - Vegetable and Chickpea Curry
Dessert - Pumpkin Pie Pudding

Day Three:

Breakfast - Blueberry Coconut Quinoa
Lunch - Vegan Chili
Dinner - Tangy Vegan Meatballs
Dessert - Creamsicle Tapioca Pudding

Day Four:

Breakfast - Strawberry Cake Oatmeal
Lunch - Butternut Squash and Applesauce
Dinner - Vegan Sausage and Bean Stew
Dessert - Apple Cobbler

Day Five:

Breakfast - Cinnamon Apple Oatmeal
Lunch - Spicy Black Bean Soup
Dinner - Vegetable Curry with Sweet Potato & Chickpeas
Dessert - Peanut Butter Chocolate Slow Cooker Cake

Day Six:

Breakfast - Almond Milk Vanilla Spice Oatmeal
Lunch - Lentil Soup
Dinner - Saag Aloo
Dessert - Rice Pudding

Day Seven:

Breakfast - Carrot Cardamom Oatmeal
Lunch - Vegan Chicken and Sweet Potato Southwestern Stew
Dinner - Lentil Bolognese
Dessert - Pumpkin Bread

7 Day Vegan Meal Plan Shopping List

Here, you will find all that you need for the 7 days' worth of meals. Non-perishable items are listed first (herbs and spices, baking goods, canned/jarred goods). Perishable ingredients are organized by day, as they will need to be purchased fresh.

Herbs and Spices:

Allspice, cumin, red pepper flakes, ground red pepper, salt, sea salt, vegetable stock cube, bay leaves, cinnamon sticks, ground cinnamon, black pepper, Italian seasoning, ground ginger, nutmeg, curry powder, mild curry paste, pumpkin pie spice, cayenne pepper, garlic powder, garlic powder, paprika, coriander, chili powder, cardamom, garam masala, hot chili powder, saffron, oregano, rosemary,

Sauces and Oils:

Olive oil, vegan margarine, coconut oil, A1 Sauce, hot pepper sauce, canola oil

Baking Goods:

Vanilla extract, steel-cut oats, rolled oats, brandy or rum, brown sugar, sugar, maple syrup, maple extract, Ener-G egg replacer, Bisquick, shredded coconut, cocoa powder, orange extract, flour, dried cranberries, dried cherries, Sucanat, baking powder, vegan chocolate chips (Trader Joe's), peanut butter, baking soda

Canned/Jarred Goods:

Vegetable stock, peeled whole tomatoes, diced fire roasted tomatoes, tomatoes with green chilies, diced Italian seasoned tomatoes, crushed tomatoes, diced tomatoes, tomato sauce, tomato paste, corn, baked beans, vegetable broth, chickpeas, pumpkin, coconut milk, black beans, pinto beans, kidney beans, chili sauce, grape jelly, fire roasted diced chili, chipotle chili in adobo sauce,

Frozen:

Corn, blueberries

Daily Fresh Purchases

Day One:

- Unsweetened almond milk
- 7 bananas
- Vanilla or coconut yogurt
- Vanilla wafers
- Baby carrots
- 16 ounces (448 g) seitan chunks
- Garlic cloves
- 3 green onions
- 2 large tomatoes
- 2 potatoes
- 1 yellow pepper
- 1 orange pepper
- 1 yellow onion
- 1 eggplant
- 1 zucchini
- 1 butternut squash
- Pecans
- White bread

Day Two:

- Unsweetened almond milk
- 1 pear
- Walnuts
- 16 oz (448 g) vegan hamburger (LightLife, Boca)
- 4 Garlic cloves
- White potatoes
- Jalapeno peppers
- Fresh ginger
- Carrots
- Green beans
- Onions
- Red potatoes

- Baby spinach
- 1 chili pepper
- Lemon
- Couscous
- Nondairy creamer

Day Three:

- Quinoa
- Almonds
- Blueberries
- Garlic cloves
- 1 red bell pepper
- 1 red onion
- 28 oz (784 g) vegan meatballs (MorningStar)
- Rice
- Lettuce
- Tomato
- Small pearl tapioca
- Almond milk

Day Four:

- Strawberries
- Almond milk
- Coconut yogurt
- 1 butternut squash
- 1 lemon
- 3 Granny Smith apples
- Red or green apples (red delicious, golden delicious, gala)
- 1 pound (450 g) vegan sausage (Light Life or MorningStar)
- Carrots
- Celery
- 2 brown potatoes
- Dried lima beans

Day Five:

- Almond milk
- Raisins
- Pecans
- Walnuts
- Apples
- Bananas
- Jalapeno peppers
- 1 pound (450 g) dry black beans
- Ginger
- Cauliflower
- Garlic cloves
- 1 medium onion
- 1 Gala apple
- 1 sweet potato
- Parsley

Day Six:

- Almond milk
- 1 vanilla bean
- Raspberries
- Blueberries
- Blackberries
- Onions
- 16 oz (448 g) bag of lentils
- Fresh spinach
- Potatoes
- Dried apricots
- Rice
- Vanilla almond milk

Day Seven:

- Carrots
- Almond milk
- Pistachios
- Pineapple juice

- 15 oz (420 g) vegan chicken (Gardein, Lifelight Chicken Strips)
- 2 large sweet potatoes
- Lentils
- Tomatoes
- 3 celery sticks
- Garlic cloves
- 1 medium onion
- 1 package of vegan noodles (any kind)
- Fresh parsley

Bonus

As a perk for purchasing this book, you can get a printable meal plan and shopping list by signing up for my newsletter at the link below:

https://gotorecipecookbooks.com/vegan-sc/

If you enjoyed the recipes in this book, please take a moment to leave a review at your favorite retailer.

Thank you for trying out this recipe cookbook.

Rachel Richards

Breakfast

For The Vegan Lifestyle

1 - Cinnamon Apple Oatmeal

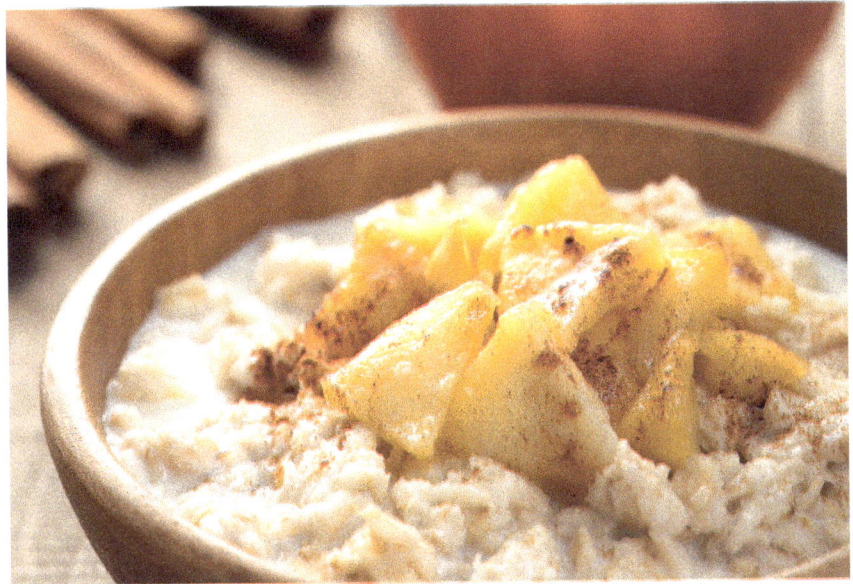

This recipe takes a classic combination to a new level. After making your own cinnamon apple oatmeal, you will never buy the microwavable version again!

Use a 2 to 3 quart (2-3 L) slow cooker.

Makes 6 to 8 servings.

Ingredients:

- ¼ teaspoon (1.25 ml) sea salt
- 1 teaspoon (5 ml) cinnamon
- 1 tablespoon (15 ml) brown sugar
- 1 tablespoon (15 ml) Sucanat
- 1 tablespoon (15 ml) coconut oil
- 1 cup (240 ml) steel-cut oats
- 1 ½ cups (360 ml) coconut or almond milk

- 1 ½ cups (360 ml) water
- 2 apples, cored, peeled, and diced

For the Toppings (optional)
- Raisins
- Pecans
- Walnuts
- Apples
- Bananas

Directions:

Spray the inside of the slow cooker with oil. Add all ingredients (except toppings) and stir. Cook on low overnight (5 to 7 hours). When finished, stir and serve, adding toppings as desired.

2 - Vanilla Fig Oatmeal

This gourmet breakfast is a delight and a treat to anyone and should be enjoyed on special occasions. It could be served as not only a breakfast, but a dessert!

Use a 1 ½ to 2 quart (1.5-2 L) slow cooker.

Makes 2 to 3 servings.

Ingredients:

- ¼ teaspoon (1.25 ml) food grade orange flower water (optional)
- ¼ teaspoon (1.25 ml) cardamom
- 1 teaspoon (5 ml) vanilla extract
- ½ cup (120 ml) chopped dried figs
- ½ cup (120 ml) steel-cut oats
- 2 cups (480 ml) unsweetened coconut milk

For the Toppings

- pinch of cinnamon
- 1 tablespoon (15 ml) chopped pistachios
- 1 tablespoon (15 ml) chopped walnuts
- 1 tablespoon (15 ml) chopped almonds
- 1 tablespoon (15 ml) brown rice syrup
- 1 tablespoon (15 ml) maple syrup

Directions:

Spray the slow cooker with oil and add all ingredients (except toppings). Allow to cook overnight on low, or 7 to 9 hours. While cooking, mix all topping ingredients in a bowl and keep in the fridge overnight. The next day, stir the oatmeal and spoon into servings. Add the topping to desired sweetness.

3 - Walnut Maple Pear Oatmeal

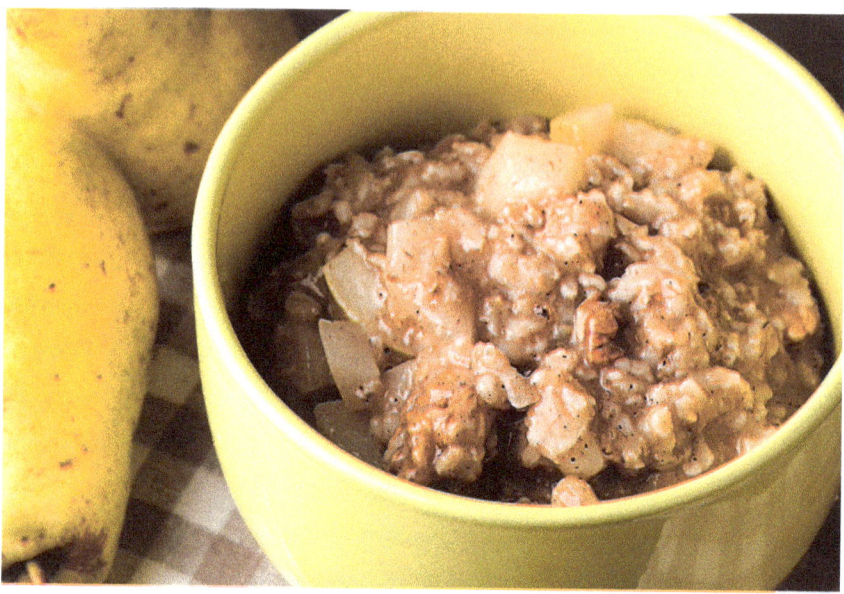

Both gluten and soy-free, this recipe will help you start your day off right. Enjoy with almond milk on top or the side, and serve warm.

Use a 1 ½ to 2 quart (1.5-2 L) slow cooker.

Makes 2 to 3 servings.

Ingredients:

- Sweetener
- ½ teaspoon (2.5 ml) vanilla extract
- ½ teaspoon (2.5 ml) maple extract
- ½ cup (120 ml) steel-cut oats
- 2 cups (480 ml) unsweetened almond milk
- 1 chopped pear

For the Toppings

- Grated nutmeg
- Maple syrup (optional)
- ¼ cup (60 ml) chopped walnuts

Directions:

First, spray a non-stick oil on the inside of the slow cooker. Add the almond milk, oats, pear, vanilla extract and maple extract. Set the temperature to low and allow to cook overnight, or 7 to 9 hours. After finished, thoroughly stir the sweetener into oatmeal. Add chopped walnuts and nutmeg as toppings. For additional sweetness, drizzle on maple syrup.

4 - Carrot Cardamom Oatmeal

Filled with nutritious ingredients, this recipe is very healthy and still delicious.

Use a 1 ½ to 2 quart (1.5-2 L) slow cooker.

Makes 2 to 3 servings.

Ingredients:

- 1 teaspoon (5 ml) ground cardamom
- 1-2 tablespoons (15-30 ml) maple syrup
- ½ cup (120 ml) steel-cut oats
- 1 cup (240 ml) shredded carrots
- 2 cups (480 ml) coconut or almond milk

For the Toppings
- Pinch of saffron
- Chopped pistachios

Directions:

Spray the slow cooker with oil. Add cardamom, oats, carrots, and nut milk. Allow to cook overnight on low, or 7 to 9 hours. When finished, stir the maple syrup into the oatmeal. Spoon the servings into bowls and top with pistachios and saffron.

5 - Strawberry Cake Oatmeal

Filled with strawberries, this recipe tastes best in the summer but may be enjoyed any time of year.

Use a 1 ½ to 2 quart (1.5-2 L) slow cooker.

Makes 2 to 3 servings.

Ingredients:

- 1 teaspoon (5 ml) vanilla extract
- 1-2 tablespoons (15-30 ml) maple syrup
- ½ cup (120 ml) steel-cut oats
- 1 cup (240 ml) chopped strawberries
- 2 cups (480 ml) unsweetened coconut or almond milk

For the Toppings
- Coconut yogurt
- Strawberries

Directions:

Spray the slow cooker with oil and place all ingredients (except sweetener and toppings) inside. Set to low and allow to cook overnight, or 7 to 9 hours. In the morning, stir in maple syrup and smash strawberries well into the mix. Spoon servings into bowls and top with the coconut yogurt and additional strawberries.

6 - Banana Pudding Oatmeal

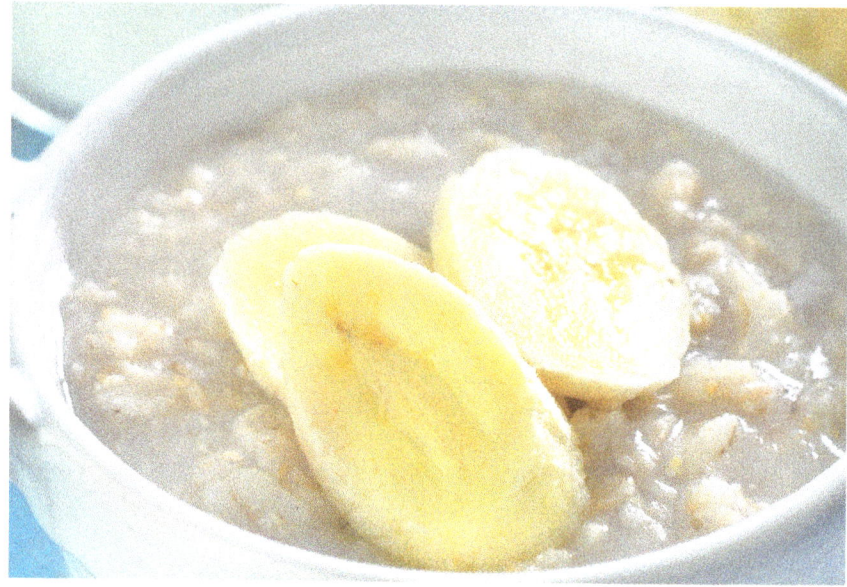

If you enjoy sweet breakfasts, but you do not enjoy the extra calories, look no further! Banana pudding oatmeal tastes like a dessert and keeps you satisfied throughout the morning.

Use a 1 ½ to 2 quart (1.5-2 L) slow cooker.

Makes 2 to 3 servings.

Ingredients:

- 1 teaspoon (5 ml) vanilla extract
- 1-2 tablespoons (15-30 ml) maple syrup
- ½ cup (120 ml) steel-cut oats
- 2 cups (480 ml) unsweetened almond milk
- 1 mashed banana

For the Toppings

- Vanilla or coconut yogurt
- Sliced bananas
- Vanilla wafers (optional)

Directions:

The night before the breakfast will be served, spread a small amount of oil on the slow cooker's base. Put the oats, almond milk, and vanilla in and allow to cook overnight on low, or 7 to 9 hours. In the morning, stir in the maple syrup and mashed banana. To serve, spoon into bowls and top with coconut yogurt and sliced bananas. For a greater treat, smash vanilla wafers and sprinkle on top.

7 - Blueberry Coconut Quinoa

Quinoa can be served as more than just dinner! The grain can also be enjoyed as a filling and wholesome breakfast. Combined with the flavors of blueberry and coconut, this breakfast recipe will become your new favorite.

Use a 2 to 3 quart (2-3 L) slow cooker.

Makes 4 servings.

Ingredients:

- 1 tablespoon (15 ml) maple syrup
- ¼ cup (60 ml) shredded coconut
- ¾ cup (180 ml) quinoa
- 1 can (13.5 oz or 400 ml) coconut milk

For the Toppings

- ¼ cup (60 ml) toasted coconut
- ¼ cup (60 ml) chopped almonds
- 2 cups (480 ml) fresh or frozen blueberries

Directions:

Spray the inside of the slow cooker with oil. Rinse the quinoa and add it to the slow cooker. Evenly sprinkle the shredded coconut to the top and drizzle maple syrup. Then open the canned coconut milk, stir and add to the slow cooker. Briefly stir all of the ingredients together and cook on low for three hours, or high for 1 ½ to 2 hours. When finished, stir and serve into four bowls. Add a tablespoon (15 ml) of toasted coconut and almonds to each, as well as ½ cup (120 ml) of blueberries.

8 - Breakfast Quinoa

Quick and easy to make, this appealing breakfast blends together an assortment of warm and sweet flavors. Serve on a chilly day, or enjoy as a comfort food any time of year.

Use a 1 ½ to 2 quart (1.5-2 L) slow cooker.

Makes 5 servings.

Ingredients:

- ¼ teaspoon (1.25 ml) salt
- ¼ teaspoon (1.25 ml) nutmeg
- 1 teaspoon (5 ml) vanilla extract
- 2 teaspoons (10 ml) cinnamon
- ¼ cup (60 ml) pepitas
- 1 cup (240 ml) quinoa
- 3 cups (720 ml) almond milk
- 1 peeled and diced apple
- 4 chopped dates

Directions:

Spray inside of the slow cooker with oil. Add all ingredients to the slow cooker and stir together. Cook on high for two hours, occasionally stirring. Or, cook on low overnight (8 hours). When finished, stir and serve!

9 - Lemon Blueberry Muffin Oatmeal

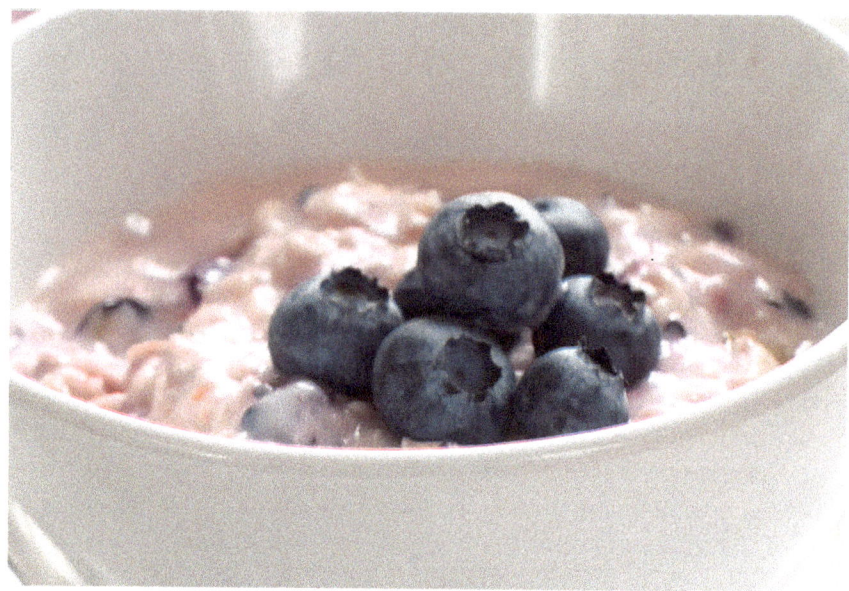

An enjoyable breakfast, this recipe's ingredients blend together into a delightful combination. Enjoy as a snack as well as a breakfast.

Use a 1 ½ to 2 quart (1.5-2 L) slow cooker.

Makes 2 to 3 servings.

Ingredients:

- ¼ teaspoon (1.25 ml) lemon extract
- 1 teaspoon (5 ml) vanilla extract
- 1-2 tablespoons (15-30 ml) maple syrup
- ½ cup (120 ml) steel-cut oats
- 1 cup (250 ml) blueberries
- 2 cups (480 ml) unsweetened coconut milk

For the Toppings
- Lemon zest
- Blueberries

Directions:

Spray the slow cooker with oil and add all ingredients (except toppings and maple syrup). Allow to cook on low overnight, or 7 to 9 hours. In the morning, stir in maple syrup and top with more blueberries and lemon zest.

10 - Almond Milk Vanilla Spice Oatmeal

This recipe contains many warm, sweet flavors and spices. Enjoy on cold days as a breakfast or dessert.

Use a 2 to 3 quart (2-3 L) slow cooker.

Makes 3 to 4 servings.

Ingredients:

- ⅛ teaspoon (0.6 ml) cardamom
- ⅛ teaspoon (0.6 ml) nutmeg
- ¼ teaspoon (1.25 ml) cinnamon
- 2 tablespoons (30 ml) brown sugar
- 1 cup (240 ml) steel-cut oats
- 1-2 cups (240-480 ml) almond milk
- 3 ½ cups (840 ml) water
- 1 vanilla bean

For the Toppings

- Raspberries
- Blueberries
- Blackberries

Directions:

Spray the inside of the slow cooker with oil. Add cardamom, nutmeg, cinnamon, vanilla bean, brown sugar, oats, and water. Cook on low overnight, or 7 to 9 hours. When finished, add almond milk to desired consistency and serve in bowls, adding toppings. For additional sweetness, stir in more brown sugar.

Soups and Stews

11 - Ratatouille

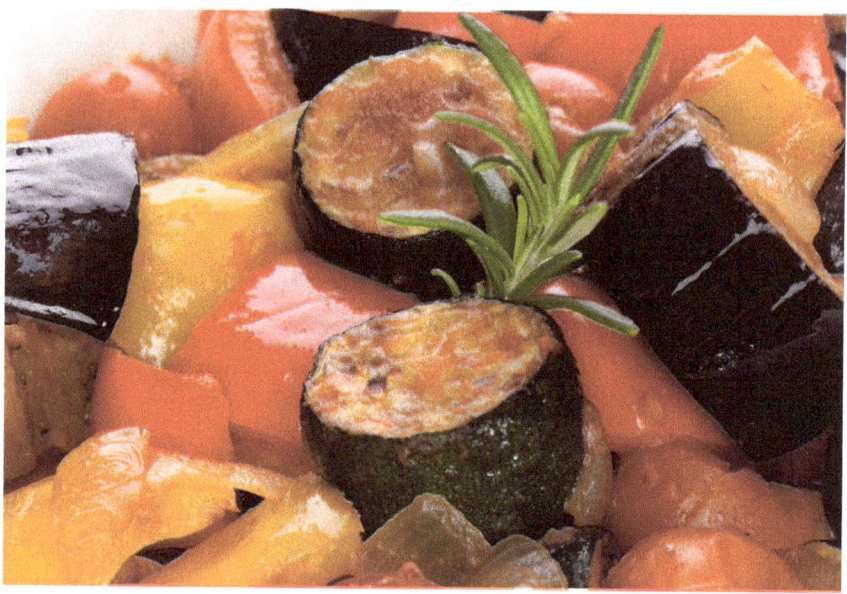

Feel like you are eating authentic Italian cuisine with this ratatouille recipe. Many Italian dishes contain meat, cheese, or both—but this recipe has neither.

Use a 4 quart (4 L) slow cooker or bigger.

Ingredients:

- ½ teaspoon (2.5 ml) black pepper
- 1 teaspoon (5 ml) salt
- 1 teaspoon (5 ml) Italian seasoning or allspice
- 2 tablespoons (30 ml) olive oil
- ½ cup (120 ml) water
- 1 can (14 oz or 392 g) peeled whole tomatoes, drained
- 1 can (14 oz or 392 g) diced fire roasted tomatoes
- 3 minced garlic cloves
- 1 yellow pepper
- 1 orange pepper
- ½ yellow onion
- 1 eggplant

- 1 zucchini
- 1 butternut squash

Directions:

Cut all vegetables and spread onto the bottom of the slow cooker in a neat arrangement (not necessary, but enjoyable). Sprinkle spices overtop and pour on oil, water, and canned tomatoes. Allow to cook for 5 to 6 hours on low, or 3 to 4 hours on high. When finished, stir and serve.

12 - Vegan Cassoulet

You can now enjoy a cassoulet without eating meat! And, you can eat a cassoulet and still stay on track.

Use a 4 quart (4 L) slow cooker.

Makes 4 servings.

Ingredients:

- salt to taste
- 1 sprig rosemary
- 2 bay leaves
- ½ teaspoon (2.5 ml) smoked paprika
- 1 teaspoon (5 ml) thyme
- 1 tablespoon (15 ml) Herbs de Provence
- 1 tablespoon (15 ml) vegan chicken bouillon
- ½ cup (120 ml) vegan sausage crumbles (such as Morning Star)
- 1 ½ cups (360 ml) vegan chicken (such as Gardein or Smart Strips)
- 1-2 cups water (240-480 ml)
- 1 ½ cups (360 ml) diced tomatoes
- 2 cups (480 ml) pre-cooked field peas or black-eyed peas
- 1 small minced onion
- 2 stalks chopped celery
- 3 small chopped carrots

Directions:

Start by sautéing the onion in a bit of water over medium heat. Then, add vegan sausage crumbles and cook until brown. Then, cut carrots and celery and store all ingredients in the fridge until morning. Spray the inside of the slow cooker with oil and add all ingredients, gently stirring. Allow to cook on low for 6 to 8 hours. After cooking is done, remove rosemary stems. Serve while hot.

13 - Spicy Black Bean Soup

Kick up your black beans a notch with this recipe. Enjoy plain, or add crackers and tortillas for a crunchy twist.

Use a 4 quart (4 L) slow cooker.

Makes 6 servings.

Ingredients:

- ½ teaspoon (2.5 ml) hot pepper sauce
- ½ teaspoon (2.5 ml) garlic powder
- ¾ teaspoon (3.75 ml) ground black pepper
- 1 teaspoon (5 ml) cayenne pepper
- 1 teaspoon (5 ml) ground cumin
- 1 tablespoon (15 ml) chili powder
- 4 teaspoons (20 ml) diced jalapeno peppers
- 6 cups (1.44 L) vegetable broth
- 1 pound (450 g) dry black beans, soaked overnight

Directions:

After the beans are finished soaking, drain and rinse them. Spray inside of slow cooker. Add all ingredients, stirring in all seasonings. Allow to cook for four hours on high, and then cook for two hours on low. When ready to eat, stir thoroughly and serve.

14 - Vegan Gumbo

If you love veggies, this recipe will be your new favorite. It combines corn, peppers, lima beans, okra, onion, and tomatoes to form a delicious and healthy soup. Enjoy with crackers or bread.

Use a 4 quart (4 L) slow cooker.

Ingredients:

- ¼ teaspoon (1.25 ml) allspice
- 1 teaspoon (5 ml) salt
- 1 cup (240 ml) corn kernels
- 1 cup (240 ml) cooked lima beans
- 1 ½ cup (360 ml) sliced okra
- 2 cups (480 ml) tomatoes, diced
- 4 cups (960 ml) vegetable stock
- 3 minced garlic cloves
- 1 diced green pepper
- 1 chopped onion

Directions:

Before adding to the slow cooker, sauté the garlic, green pepper, and onion in a pan on medium heat with water. Remove garlic cloves and place all ingredients in the slow cooker. Allow to cook for 6 hours on high, or 8 to 10 hours on low while stirring occasionally. After finished, stir one last time and serve.

15 - Farro and Veggie Split Pea Soup

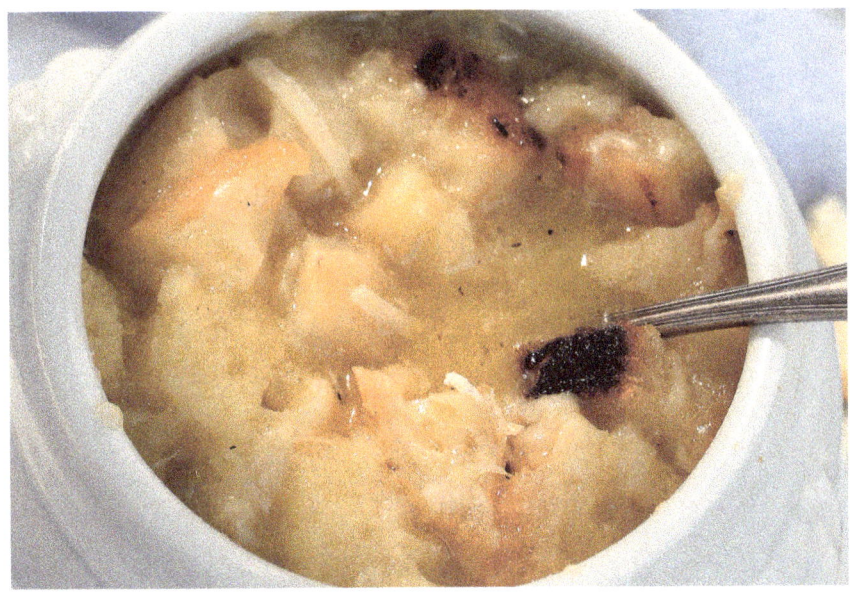

This recipe is very healthy and filled with beneficial ingredients. Farro is a grain rich in nutrients and works great for soup.

Use a 4 quart (4 L) slow cooker.

Makes 6 to 8 servings.

Ingredients:

- 2 veggie bouillon cubes
- 3 bay leaves
- 1 teaspoon (5 ml) turmeric
- 2 teaspoons (10 ml) garam masala
- 2 teaspoons (10 ml) smoked paprika
- 1 cup (240 ml) split peas
- 1 ½ cups (360 ml) farro
- 2 cups (480 ml) chopped potato or turnip
- 8 cups (1.92 L) water

- Salt and pepper to taste

Directions:

Spray the inside of the slow cooker with oil. Add all ingredients and stir. Then, cook on low for 8 to 10 hours, or on high for 3 to 4 hours. When finished, stir and serve, adding salt and pepper to taste. Additional water may be mixed in for a thinner consistency.

16 - Vegan Greek Stew

Most Greek dishes are not vegan-friendly. Enjoy the cuisine of the Mediterranean without the meat and cheese.

Use a 3 to 4 quart (3-4 L) slow cooker.

Ingredients:

- ¼ teaspoon (1.25 ml) pepper
- ½ teaspoon (2.5 ml) salt
- ½ teaspoon (2.5 ml) allspice
- 1 teaspoon (5 ml) cumin
- ½ cup (120 ml) vegan or tofu feta cheese (VegCuisine Soy Feta Cheese)
- 1 cup (240 ml) chopped zucchini
- 2 cups (480 ml) butternut squash
- 2 cups (480 ml) chopped carrots
- 14 oz can (420 ml) vegetable broth
- 15 oz can (420 g) rinsed and drained garbanzo beans
- 2 cans (14 oz or 392 g each) undrained diced tomatoes
- 4 cups (960 ml) hot cooked couscous
- 2 minced garlic cloves
- 2 chopped onions

Directions:

Mix all ingredients in slow cooker except for feta cheese and couscous. Allow to cook for 7 to 9 hours on low. When finished, serve with couscous and sprinkled feta cheese.

17 - Lentil Soup

A quick and easy recipe, lentil soup makes an appetizing lunch. Serve with toast or crackers, or enjoy as a side dish.

Use a 4 quart (4 L) slow cooker.

Ingredients:

- ½ cup (120 ml) onion
- 1 can (8 oz or 240 ml) vegetable broth
- 1 large can (28 oz or 784 g) crushed tomatoes
- 16 oz (448 g) bag of lentils

Directions:

Add all ingredients to the slow cooker and fill with water. Allow to cook for about 8 hours and serve.

18 - Eggplant and Tomato Garbanzo Bean Stew

This recipe is best served in the summer with fresh produce and spices. Try serving with a salad as a side.

Use a 3 ½ to 5 quart (3.5-5 L) slow cooker.

Makes 6 servings.

Ingredients:

- ¼ teaspoon (1.25 ml) salt
- ¼ teaspoon (1.25 ml) pepper
- ¼ teaspoon (1.25 ml) crushed red pepper
- ½ teaspoon (2.5 ml) dried oregano
- ½ teaspoon (2.5 ml) dried basil
- 6 ounces (180 ml) tomato paste
- 1 cup (240 ml) chopped onion
- 1 cup (240 ml) sliced celery
- 8 ounce (240 ml) can kidney beans, drained
- 1 ½ cups (360 ml) sliced carrot
- 15 ounce can (450 ml) drained garbanzo beans
- 2 cups (480 ml) chopped tomato
- 3 cups (720 ml) vegetable broth
- 1 bay leaf
- 3 minced garlic cloves
- 1 medium peeled eggplant

Directions:

Place the onion, celery, garlic, carrot, kidney beans, tomato, garbanzo beans, and eggplant in the slow cooker. In a bowl, mix the rest of the ingredients. Stir and pour into the slow cooker over the vegetables. Allow to cook for 7 to 8 hours on low, or 3 ½ to 4 hours on high.

19 - Vegan Pumpkin Chicken Chowder

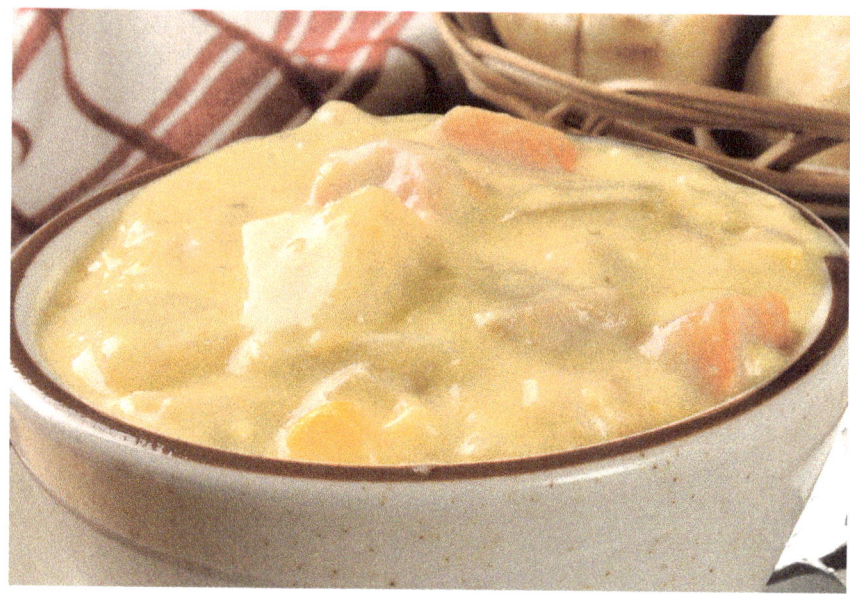

This recipe contains a surprisingly good combination: pumpkin and chicken (not real chicken, of course). With corn and spices added, Vegan Pumpkin Chicken Chowder is sure to be a crowd-pleaser.

Use a 4 quart (4 L) slow cooker.

Ingredients:

- Cayenne or chipotle powder to taste
- Salt and pepper to taste
- 1 bay leaf
- 2 minced cloves garlic
- 2 sprigs fresh thyme or 1 teaspoon (5 ml) dried
- 1 tablespoon (15 ml) vegan chicken bouillon
- ½ cup (120 ml) pumpkin purée
- 1 cup (240 ml) corn kernels (fresh or frozen)
- 1 cup (240 ml) unsweetened almond milk
- 1 ½ cups (360 ml) vegan chicken (such as Gardein or Smart Strips)
- 4 cups (960 ml) water
- 1 medium diced potato

Directions:

Prepare ingredients by cutting vegan chicken and all other vegetables. Allow puree to thaw. Combine ingredients and keep in the refrigerator overnight. In the morning, add all ingredients, excluding the milk, to the slow cooker. Also add salt and pepper if desired. Allow to cook on low for 6 to 8 hours, or on high for 3 to 4 hours. When finished, remove the bay leaf and fresh thyme sprigs before adding almond milk. Mix thoroughly. Taste the chowder and add cayenne pepper, salt and pepper if necessary.

20 - Black Beans and Rice Soup

This recipe is ideal for vegans and vegetarians who struggle to find protein sources. Its medley of flavors and ingredients are delicious for both vegans and non-vegans.

Use a 4 quart (4 L) slow cooker.

Makes 8 servings.

Ingredients:

- ½ teaspoon (2.5 ml) chili powder
- ½ teaspoon (2.5 ml) dried oregano
- ½ teaspoon (2.5 ml) Tabasco sauce
- ½ teaspoon (2.5 ml) ground cumin
- 1 ½ teaspoon (7.5 ml) dried basil
- 1 ½ cups (360 ml) cooked rice
- 14 ½ oz can (435 ml) crushed tomatoes
- 2 x 14 ½ oz cans (435 ml each) vegetable broth
- 2 x 16 oz cans (480 ml each) drained and rinsed black beans
- 2 stalks thinly sliced celery
- 4 minced garlic cloves
- 3 thinly sliced carrots
- 1 medium chopped onion

Directions:

Excluding the rice, combine all ingredients in the slow cooker. Allow to cook for 8 to 10 hours on low, or 3 to 4 hours on high. Add heated cooked rice before serve.

21 - Black Bean-Chipotle Chili

This chili recipe is perfect for any cold day and is a great protein source. Packed with flavor, it is delicious for dinner or lunch.

Use a 4 quart (4 L) slow cooker.

Makes 6 servings.

Ingredients:

- Salt to taste
- ½ teaspoon (2.5 ml) ground cumin
- ½ teaspoon (2.5 ml) chipotle pepper powder
- 1 teaspoon (5 ml) minced garlic
- 1 tablespoon (15 ml) chili powder
- ¼ cup (60 ml) chopped fresh cilantro (optional)
- ½ cup (120 ml) chopped onion
- 1 cup (240 ml) salsa
- 2 x 14.5 oz cans (406 g each) undrained diced tomatoes with green peppers & onions
- 2 x 15 oz cans (420 g) rinsed & drained black beans

Directions:

Add all ingredients to the slow cooker, except cilantro. Allow to cook on low for 6 to 8 hours. When finished, add cilantro and stir. Serve while hot.

22 - Navy Bean Soup

A recipe perfect for any meal, navy bean soup is packed with health benefits and flavor. Try serving with a salad or freshly made bread.

Use a 4 quart (4 L) slow cooker or bigger.

Makes 2 servings.

Ingredients:

- dash of crushed red pepper
- ⅓ bay leaf
- ⅛ teaspoon (0.6 ml) thyme
- ⅓ teaspoon (1.7 ml) paprika
- 1 teaspoon (5 ml) garlic powder
- ⅛ cup (30 ml) chopped onions
- ⅓ pound (150 g) dried navy beans
- 10 oz (280 g) canned vegetable broth
- 10 oz (280 g) canned diced tomatoes

Directions:

Soak the beans overnight, then rinse and drain in the morning. Add all ingredients to the slow cooker. Pour enough water over the mixture to cover by an inch. Allow to cook for 4 hours on low and serve.

23 - Bean Stew

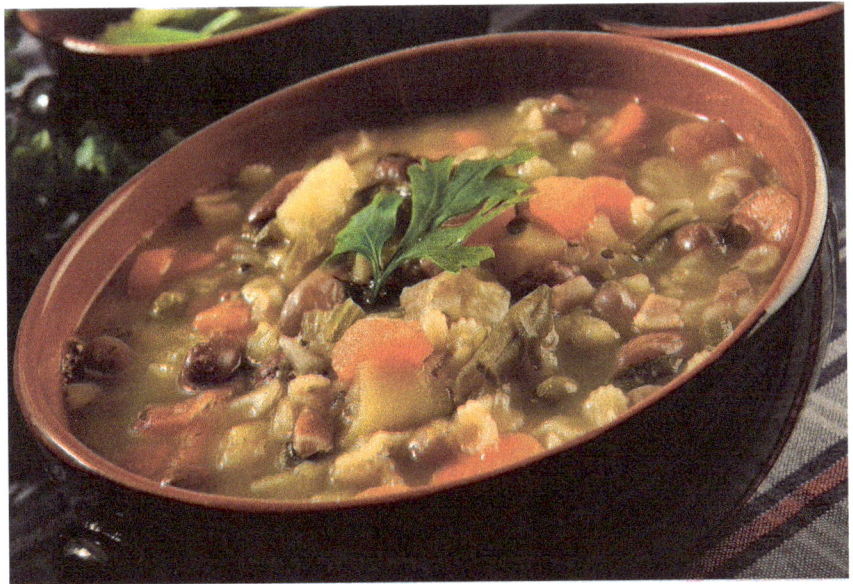

This recipe is filled with vegetables that provides essential nutrients and keeps you full. Serve this bean stew as a side or as an appetizer.

Use a 6 quart (6 L) slow cooker.

Ingredients:

- ½ teaspoon (2.5 ml) black pepper
- 1 teaspoon (5 ml) dill
- 1 teaspoon (5 ml) salt
- 1 ½ teaspoons (7.5 ml) paprika
- 1 cup (240 ml) carrots
- 2 cups (480 ml) split peas or lentils
- 1 can (15 oz or 420 g) rinsed kidney beans
- 1 can (15 oz or 420 g) rinsed black beans
- 6 cups (1.44 L) vegetable broth

- handful of broccoli (or any other desired vegetable)
- 1 chopped yellow bell pepper
- 1 chopped potato
- 3 chopped tomatoes
- 4 chopped green onions

Directions:

Rinse beans and place in the slow cooker with chopped vegetables and split peas. Pour in broth and add spices. Thoroughly stir and cook for 7 to 9 hours on low, or for 4-5 hours on high.

24 - Black Bean Soup

Enjoy this soup as a nacho dip or as a meal. It tastes great with toasted bread or a sandwich.

Use a 4 quart (4 L) slow cooker.

Ingredients:

- ½ teaspoon (2.5 ml) ground black pepper
- 1-2 teaspoon (5-10 ml) salt
- 1 teaspoon (5 ml) smoked paprika
- 2 teaspoons (10 ml) ground cumin
- 1 tablespoon (15 ml) adobo sauce
- 2 tablespoons (30 ml) lime juice
- 1 lb (450 g) dry black beans
- 4-6 cups (960 to 1,440 ml) vegetable broth
- 1 diced onion
- 2 minced chipotle peppers
- 2 diced bell peppers
- 4 minced garlic cloves

For the Toppings
- Sour cream
- Cilantro
- Tortilla chips
- Jalapenos

Directions:

Soak the beans overnight, then drain and rinse the next morning. Place beans in slow cooker and add 4 cups of vegetable broth. Cook on low heat. Sauté onions and bell peppers in a pan on medium heat and add to slow cooker when finished. Stir in garlic, adobo sauce, cumin, and paprika. Allow to cook for 7 to 8 hours on low, or for 3 to 4 hours on high. When finished, add lime juice, salt and pepper. Serve with toppings as desired.

25 - Vegan Ethiopian Chicken Stew

Enjoy an exotic cuisine right in your own home! This foreign dish is 100% vegan with replacements for chicken, butter, and eggs. Even better, it tastes great!

Use a 6 quart (6 L) slow cooker.

Makes 8 servings.

Ingredients:

- ½ teaspoon (2.5 ml) black pepper
- 1 teaspoon (5 ml) ground ginger
- 1 teaspoon (5 ml) cayenne pepper
- 1 teaspoon (5 ml) ground turmeric
- 1 tablespoon (15 ml) paprika
- 2 tablespoons (30 ml) coconut oil
- ¼ cup (60 ml) fresh lemon juice
- 1 can (14.5 oz or 406 g) undrained diced tomatoes
- 2 cups (480 ml) water
- 2 cups (480 ml) cooked cubed tofu
- 5 cups (1,200 ml) vegan chicken (such as Gardein or Smart Strips)
- 3 large diced onions

Directions:

Add tomatoes, vegan chicken, and lemon juice to slow cooker and stir. Then add all ingredients (except tofu) and pour water into the cooker. Allow to cook for 6 to 8 hours on low, or 4 to 5 hours on high. Dollop ¼ cup of tofu in each serving.

26 - Azorean Vegan Stew

Enjoy this zesty stew for a flavorful lunch or a light dinner. Use fresh vegetables and seasonings for the best taste.

Use a 4 to 6 quart (4-6 L) slow cooker.

Ingredients:

- 1 teaspoon (5 ml) allspice
- 1 teaspoon (5 ml) cumin
- ½ tablespoon (7.5 ml) red pepper flakes
- 1 tablespoon (15 ml) salt
- 1 cup (240 ml) baby carrots
- 16 ounces (448 g) seitan chunks
- 3 cups (720 ml) vegetable stock
- 1 bay leaf
- 2 cinnamon sticks
- 5-6 smashed and chopped garlic cloves
- 3 chopped green onions
- 2 large chopped tomatoes
- 2 potatoes, chopped in 1 inch (2.5 cm) chunks

Directions:

Add seitan to the slow cooker first. Pour the broth over top, and add all chopped vegetables. Stir in the rest of the seasonings and add cinnamon sticks. Allow to cook on low for 8 to 10 hours, or on high for 6 hours.

27 - Vegan Chicken and Sweet Potato Southwestern Stew

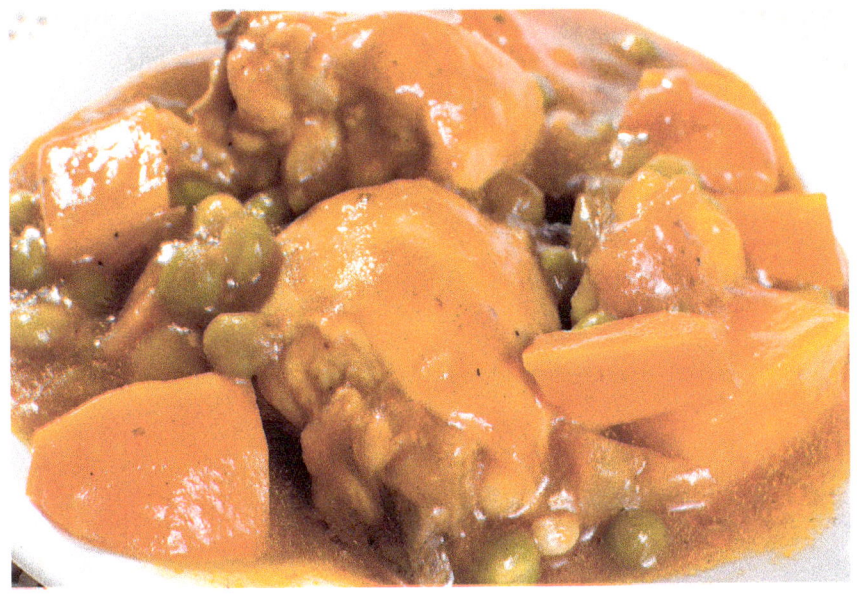

This recipe is high in protein and has a variety of harmonious flavors. Enjoy by itself or as a side dish for dinner or lunch.

Use a 4 quart (4 L) slow cooker.

Ingredients:

- 1 can (4 oz or 112 g) fire roasted diced chili
- ½ cup (120 ml) pineapple juice
- 1 can (6 ounce, 170 g) tomato paste
- 15 oz (420 g) vegan chicken (Gardein, Lifelight Chicken Strips)
- 1 can (15 oz or 420 g) plain baked beans
- 2 large peeled and cut sweet potatoes

Directions:

First, add vegan chicken and sweet potato slices. Pour the cans of baked beans, tomato paste, and diced chili over the chicken. Last, add pineapple juice. Allow the meal to cook for 6 to 8 hours on low, or for 4 hours on high. Stir and serve.

28 - Vegan Cowboy Stew

Vegans can enjoy western food, too! Make this meal when you are craving meat, or just want to spice it up.

Use a 5 quart (5 L) slow cooker or bigger.

Ingredients:

- 1 can (8 oz or 224 g) tomato sauce
- 1 cup (240 ml) water
- 1 can (14 oz or 392 g) tomatoes with green chilies
- 1 can (14.5 oz or 406 g) diced Italian seasoned tomatoes
- 1 can (15 oz or 420 g) drained corn
- 1 can (15 oz or 420 g) plain baked beans
- 16 oz (448 g) vegan hamburger (LightLife, Boca)
- 2 chopped garlic cloves
- 3 peeled and cut potatoes
- Sliced jalapeno peppers (optional)

Directions:

Before using the vegan hamburger, brown it first with the garlic and let cool before using. Drain canned corn and add to the slow cooker. Pour in other cans and combine all contents, liquid and all. Add the browned vegan hamburger and one cup (240 ml) water. Stir all ingredients together, and allow to cook for 8 to 10 hours on low, or 4 to 5 hours on high. When finished, stir and top with peppers for serving.

29 - Vegan Lamb Tagine

Enjoy this delicacy without the meat or the hassle. Eat with grains and potatoes for a filling and delicious dinner.

Use a 6 quart (6 L) slow cooker.

Ingredients:

- 1 teaspoon (5 ml) coriander
- 2 teaspoon (10 ml) ground cumin
- 2-4 tablespoon (30-60 ml) capers
- 1 head of garlic, broken into cloves
- 2 yellow onions, sliced in rings
- 2 cans (6 oz or 170 g each) drained black olives
- 1 bottle (25 oz or 750 ml) red wine
- 2 pounds (90 g) vegan lamb meat or beef, cut into chunks
- 1 inch (2.5 cm) ginger, peeled and grated

Directions:

Add cut onions and garlic cloves to the bottom of the slow cooker. Next, add the vegan meat and dust spices over the top. Mix in olives and capers, and pour the wine overtop. Allow to cook for 8 to 12 hours on low.

30 - Vegan Sausage and Bean Stew

This recipe is yet another that is packed with protein and vegetables, a great combination for healthy living. Enjoy with vegetables on the side, such as broccoli or a salad.

Use a 6 quart (6 L) slow cooker.

Ingredients:

- 1 tablespoon (15 ml) A1 Sauce
- 1 pound (450 g) vegan sausage (Light Life or MorningStar)
- 1 cup (240 ml) chopped carrot
- 1 cup (240 ml) chopped celery
- 2 diced brown potatoes
- ½ cup (120 ml) dried lima beans
- 4 cups (960 ml) vegetable broth

Directions:

Chop vegetables and add all ingredients to the slow cooker. Crumble the sausage as it is added. Cook for 8 hours on low.

Main Dishes

31 - Saag Aloo

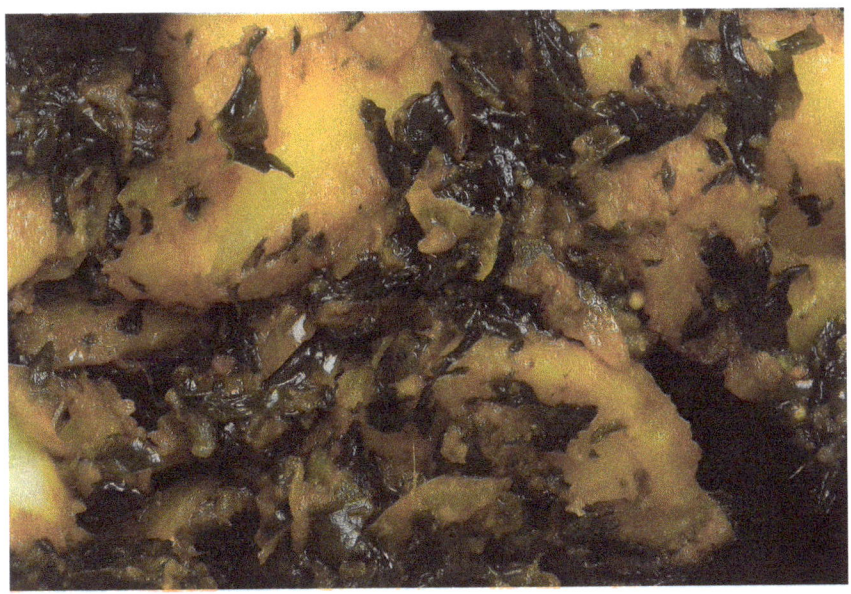

Saag Aloo is filled with spices and has a rich aroma. It takes moments for the preparation but will taste like it took hours to make!

Use a 3 ½ quart (3.5 L) slow cooker or bigger.

Ingredients:

- Black pepper
- ½ teaspoon (2.5 ml) cumin
- ½ teaspoon (2.5 ml) ground coriander
- ½ teaspoon (2.5 ml) garam masala
- ½ teaspoon (2.5 ml) hot chili powder
- 1 tablespoon (15 ml) oil
- ¼ cup (60 ml) water
- 1 cup (250 ml) fresh spinach, chopped
- 1 ½ lbs (675 g) potatoes
- ½ crumbled vegetable stock cube

- ½ thinly sliced onion

Directions:

Prepare the potatoes by peeling and cutting into 1-inch (2.5 cm) pieces. Combine potatoes in the slow cooker with all the spices, oil, stock cube, water, and onion. Add the spinach to the top, as much as desired. Allow to cook for 3 hours on medium, stirring every hour. Cooking is done when the potatoes becomes soft.

32 - Vegan "Soda Pop" Meatballs

This recipe can be used in countless ways! Serve on sandwiches, pasta, rice, and many more.

Use a 3 ½ to 4 quart (3.5-4 L) slow cooker.

Ingredients:

- 2 teaspoons (10 ml) soy sauce
- 1 can soda
- ½ jar apricot jelly
- 1 bottle steak sauce (Heinz 57, A1)
- 1 bag frozen vegan, gluten free meatballs

Directions:

Put meatballs in the slow cooker and mix other ingredients in a bowl. Add the mixture to the slow cooker and stir. Allow to cook on high for 2 to 3 hours.

33 - Vegetable and Chickpea Curry

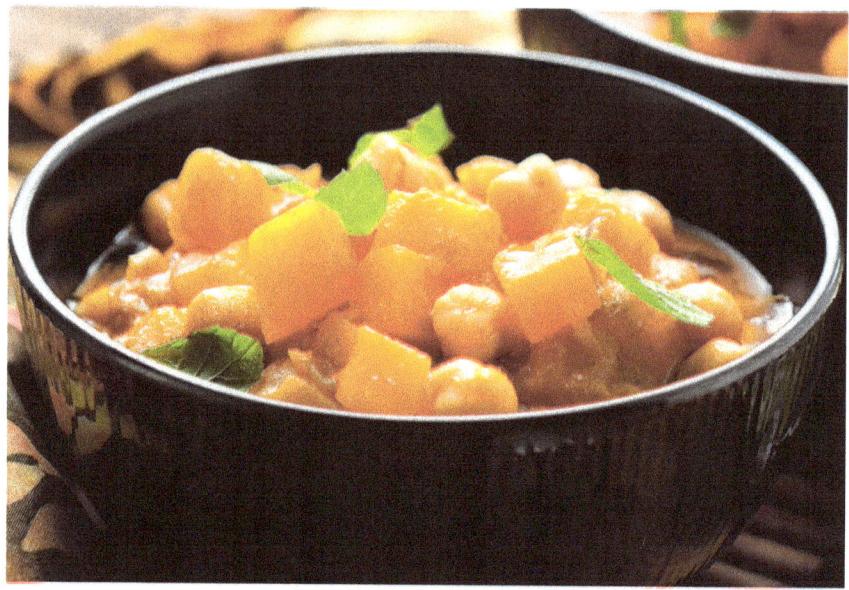

Use this recipe for a healthy, cheap, and easy meal. Use frozen or fresh vegetables, depending on the season or preference.

Use a 5 to 6 quart (5-6 L) slow cooker.

Ingredients:

- ⅛ teaspoon (0.6 ml) ground red pepper
- ¼ teaspoon (1.25 ml) pepper
- ½ teaspoon (2.5 ml) salt
- 1 teaspoon (5 ml) fresh grated ginger
- 1 teaspoon (5 ml) brown sugar
- 1 tablespoon (15 ml) olive oil
- 1 tablespoon (15 ml) curry powder
- 1 cup (240 ml) sliced carrot
- 1 cup (240 ml) cut green beans
- 1 cup (240 ml) light coconut milk
- 1 ½ cups (360 ml) chopped onion
- 1 ½ cups (360 ml) cubed red potatoes
- 1 can (14 oz or 392 g) vegetable broth
- 1 can (14.5 oz or 406 g) undrained diced tomatoes

- 3 cups (720 ml) baby spinach
- 2 cans (14 oz or 392 g each) drained chickpeas
- 2 minced garlic cloves
- 1 chili pepper

For the Toppings
- Lemon wedges
- Couscous

Directions:

Sauté the onion and carrot in oil on medium heat. After finished, add the chili pepper, garlic, ginger, sugar, and curry powder and stir to mix. Allow to cook for another 60 seconds and add to the slow cooker. Add the chickpeas with the other ingredients (except coconut milk and spinach) and the vegetable broth. Allow to cook on high for about 6 hours, and then stir in coconut milk and spinach. Serve with couscous and vegetable wedges if desired.

34 - Homemade Applesauce

Tastes even better than your grandma's! Enjoy warm or cold, as breakfast or a snack.

Use a 4 quart (4 L) slow cooker.

Ingredients:

- ½ teaspoon (2.5 ml) cinnamon
- ¼ cup (60 ml) brown sugar
- Juice from ½ lemon
- 3 peeled tart apples (Granny Smith)
- 3 peeled red or green apples (red delicious, golden delicious, gala)

Directions:

Peel and core all apples, and cut each into about 8 pieces. Place all apples in the slow cooker and squeeze lemon juice over apples. Add the measured cinnamon and brown sugar. Allow to cook on high for 2 to 3 hours (or until apples are soft and broken), occasionally stirring. May be stored in an airtight container in the refrigerator for up to ten days.

35 - Lentil Bolognese

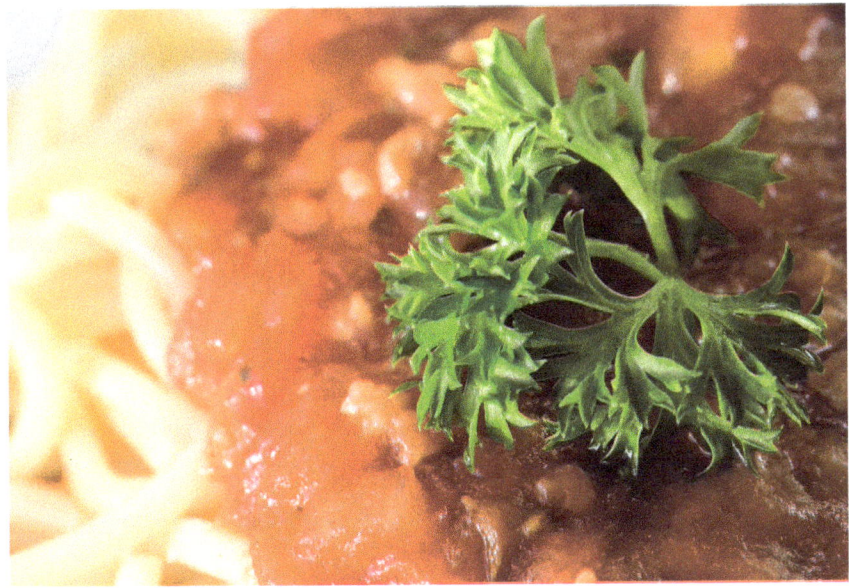

This recipe provides a meal that is a satisfying and quick dinner. Try serving with a side salad and bread.

Use a 4 quart (4 L) slow cooker or bigger.

Ingredients:

- 1 teaspoon (5 ml) ground black pepper
- 1 teaspoon (5 ml) oregano
- 1 teaspoon (5 ml) rosemary
- 1 teaspoon (5 ml) olive oil
- 1 cup (240 ml) lentils
- 1 ½ cups (360 ml) tomato puree
- 2 cups (480 ml) vegetable stock
- 1 minced chipotle chili in adobo sauce
- 2 chopped carrots
- 3 sticks chopped celery

- 4 minced garlic cloves
- 1 finely chopped medium onion
- 1 package of vegan noodles (any kind)

For the Toppings
- Salt to taste
- Fresh parsley for garnish

Directions:

Allow the lentils to soak in water while preparing. In the slow cooker, add the oil, carrots, celery, onion, garlic, a pinch of salt (optional), and half of the black pepper. Stir well and allow to cook for 30 minutes on high. Then, remove the lid and add the rest of the ingredients, including the lentils. Allow to cook for another 2 hours on high. Cook the noodles, following the directions provided, and stir into the slow cooker when finished.

36 - Vegetable Curry with Sweet Potato & Chickpeas

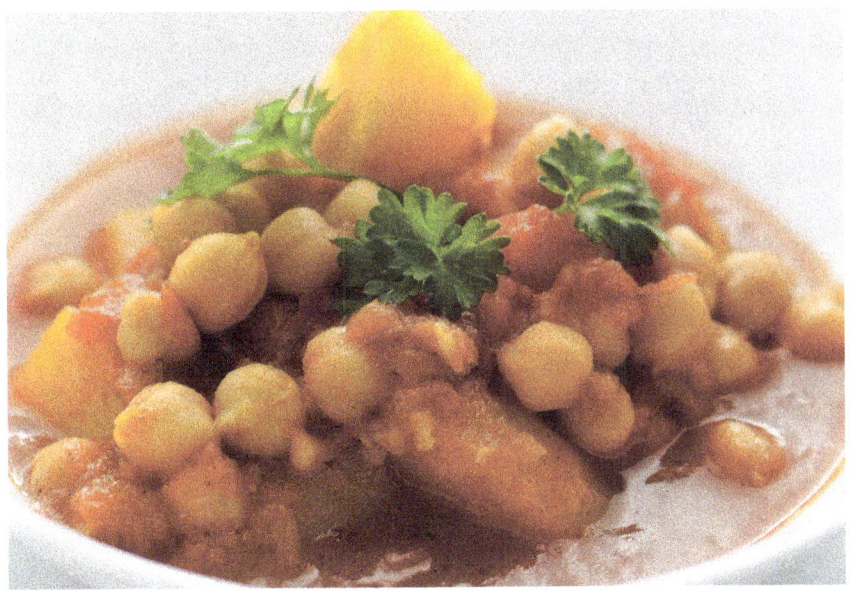

Curry puts a flavorful twist on classic sweet potato and chickpeas. Add more vegetables for an even healthier meal!

Use a 4 quart (4 L) slow cooker.

Ingredients:

- ¼ teaspoon (1.25 ml) salt
- ½ teaspoon (2.5 ml) ground pepper
- 1 teaspoon (5 ml) canola oil
- 2 tablespoons (30 ml) minced ginger
- ¼ cup (60 ml) mild curry paste (Patak's)
- ½ cup (120 ml) coconut milk
- 1 can (14 oz or 392 g) petite diced tomatoes
- 1 can (14 oz or 392 g) vegetable broth
- 2 cups (480 ml) small cauliflower florets

- 2 ½ cups (600 ml) chickpeas
- 2 minced garlic cloves
- ½ medium diced onion
- 1 diced Gala apple
- 1 peeled and cut sweet potato
- Parsley for garnish

Directions:

Sauté the ginger, onion, and apple in the canola oil on medium heat until soft. When finished, stir in garlic and curry paste for about 3 minutes, and add to the slow cooker. Add cauliflower, chickpeas, sweet potato, tomatoes, and vegetable broth. Allow to cook on high for 6 hours. After fully cooked, stir in the coconut milk. Garnish with parsley and serve.

37 - Butternut Squash

Another easy recipe, this butternut squash has only two ingredients and tastes great on sandwiches, salad, pastas, and countless more dishes. Add spices and flavorings for an extra dimension of flavor!

Use a 2 ½ to 3 quart (2.5-3 L) slow cooker.

Ingredients:

- 2-3 tablespoons (30-45 ml) water
- 1 butternut squash

Directions:

Cut the squash in halves and remove the seeds. Cut the pieces again to quarter them before placing all the pieces in the slow cooker. Add water and allow to cook on low for 3 hours. When finished, spoon out the pulp for use in your favorite dishes.

38 - Tangy Vegan Meatballs

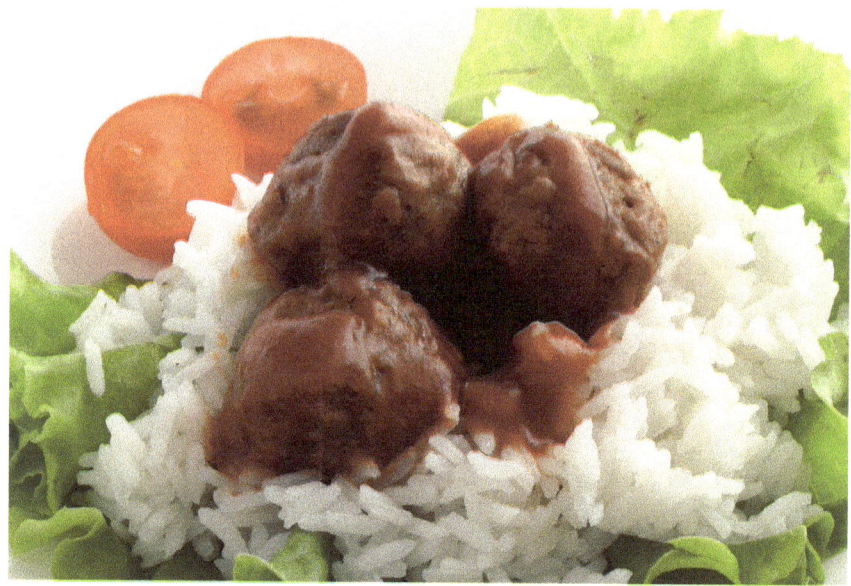

These vegan meatballs take only 2 minutes of preparation! They are incredibly easy to make and taste absolutely delicious with anything.

Use a 3 quart (3 L) slow cooker or bigger.

Ingredients:

- 12 oz jar (336 g) of chili sauce
- 18 oz jar (504 g) grape jelly
- 28 oz (784 g) vegan meatballs (MorningStar)
- Cooked rice
- Lettuce and tomato for garnish

Directions:

Combine the three ingredients in the slow cooker and allow to cook for 3 to 4 hours on low. Serve on rice and garnish with lettuce and tomato.

39 - Chipotle Style Black Beans

This recipe is simple, packed with protein, and very tasty. Eat by itself or as a dip for tortilla chips.

Use a 4 quart (4 L) slow cooker.

Ingredients:

- ¼ teaspoon (1.25 ml) black ground pepper
- 1 pound (450 g) black beans
- bay leaf
- salt to taste
- dash of ground chipotle pepper
- 2 garlic cloves
- ½ onion

Directions:

Allow the black beans to soak overnight. In the morning, drain and rinse the black beans and place in the slow cooker. Add all ingredients and enough water to cover by ½ inch (1.25 cm). Cook for 8 hours on high. When finished, stir and serve!

40 - Vegan Chili

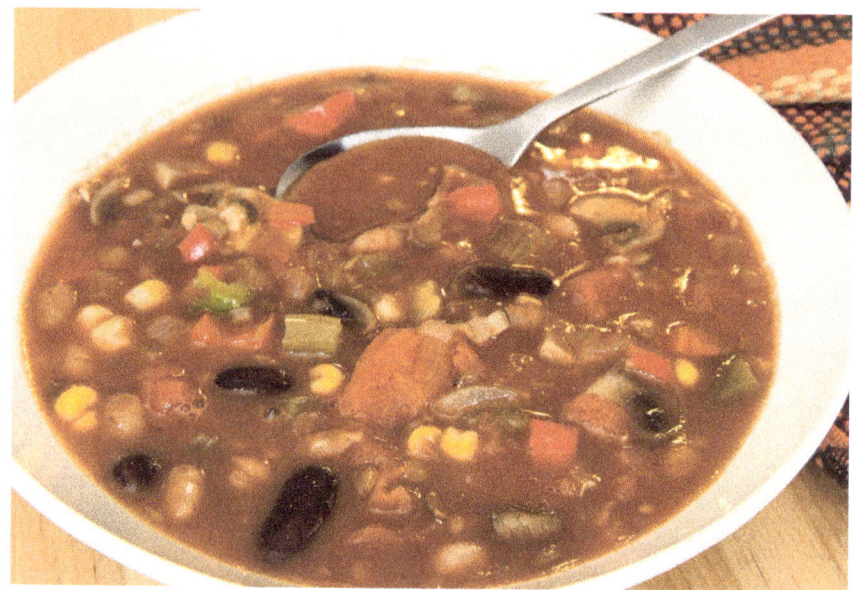

With few preparations, this recipe is easy to throw together into a slow cooker for a quick dinner! Enjoy as a soup, or as a dip for tortilla chips.

Use a 4 quart (4 L) slow cooker.

Ingredients:

- ¼ teaspoon (1.25 ml) cayenne pepper
- ½ teaspoon (2.5 ml) garlic powder
- ½ teaspoon (2.5 ml) salt
- ½ teaspoon (2.5 ml) smoked paprika
- ½ teaspoon (2.5 ml) regular paprika
- 1 teaspoon (5 ml) cumin
- 1 teaspoon (5 ml) coriander
- 1 teaspoon (5 ml) cocoa powder
- 1 tablespoon (15 ml) chili powder
- 1 cup (240 ml) fresh or frozen corn
- 1 can (15 oz or 420 g) drained and rinsed dry soaked black beans

- 1 can (15 oz or 420 g) drained and rinsed dry soaked pinto beans
- 1 can (15 oz or 420 g) drained and rinsed dry soaked kidney beans
- 2 cups (480 ml) vegetable broth
- 1 can (28 oz or 784 g) crushed tomatoes
- 5-8 minced garlic cloves
- 1 diced red bell pepper
- 1 diced red onion

Directions:

Simply combine all ingredients in your slow cooker and allow to cook for 6 to 8 hours on high.

Desserts

41 - Poached Pears In Caramel Sauce

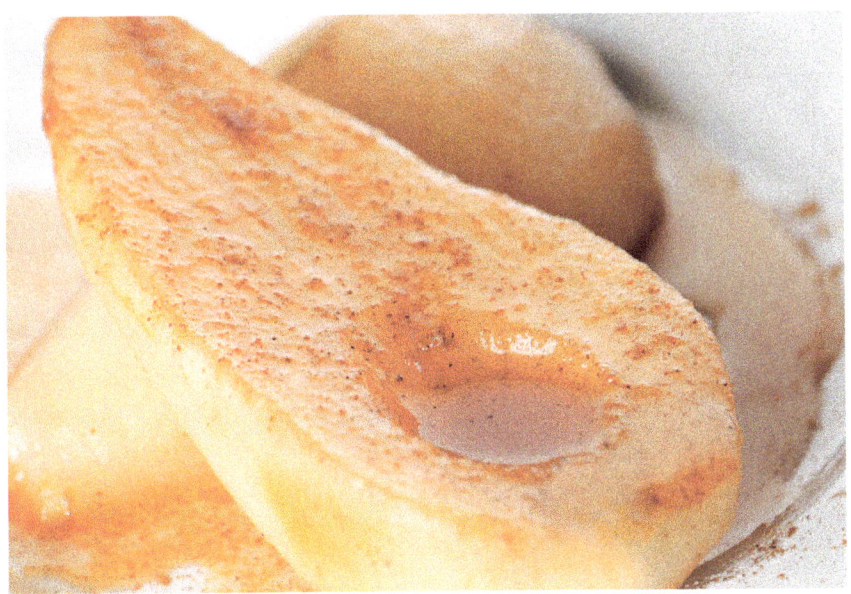

Rather than making apple dessert, try preparing a pear dessert! Pears are juicy and delicious—and taste great cooked.

Use a 4 quart (4 L) slow cooker.

Ingredients:

- ⅛ teaspoon (0.6 ml) ground cinnamon for garnish
- 1 tablespoon (15 ml) grated ginger
- 2 tablespoons (30 ml) vegan margarine
- 1 ½ cups (360 ml) brown sugar
- 4 chopped pears

Directions:

Stir ginger, margarine and brown sugar in the slow cooker. Peel and cut the pears in half. Remove the core and place pears in the slow cooker. Ensure the pears are coated with the sugar mixture. Layer the pears with the cut side done and allow to cook on high for 2 hours. After done cooking, spoon pears into a bowl and pour the liquid mixture into a sauce pan. Allow to boil and reduce heat to a simmer while stirring constantly. Once the sauce is reduced by a third of its original volume, it is ready. Spoon the caramel sauce over the pears to serve and sprinkle with cinnamon.

42 - Peanut Butter Chocolate Slow Cooker Cake

Combine two of the tastiest ingredients into one amazing dessert: chocolate and peanut butter.

Use a 3 ½ to 4 quart (3.5-4 L) slow cooker.

Makes 8 servings.

Ingredients:

For the Chocolate Layer
- 1 teaspoon (5 ml) vanilla
- 1 ½ teaspoons (7.5 ml) baking powder
- 2 tablespoons (30 ml) cocoa powder
- 2 tablespoons (30 ml) melted vegan margarine
- ½ cup (120 ml) sugar
- ½ cup (120 ml) almond milk
- ¾ cup (180 ml) vegan chocolate chips (Trader Joe's)
- 1 cup (240 ml) flour

For the Peanut Butter Layer
- ¼ cup (60 ml) cocoa powder
- ½ cup (120 ml) peanut butter
- ¾ cup (180 ml) sugar
- 1 cup (240 ml) water

Directions:

First, grease the slow cooker with oil. Start by making the chocolate layer. In a bowl, mix the baking powder, cocoa powder, sugar and flour. Then add vanilla, margarine and almond milk and stir. Lastly, mix in the chocolate chips and pour in the slow cooker.

For the peanut butter layer, mix the cocoa powder and sugar together. Boil the water and mix with peanut butter in a second bowl. Add the peanut butter mixture into the dry ingredients. Slowly and carefully pour over the chocolate batter in the slow cooker. Allow to cook for 2 to 2 ½ hours on high.

43 - Creamsicle Tapioca Pudding

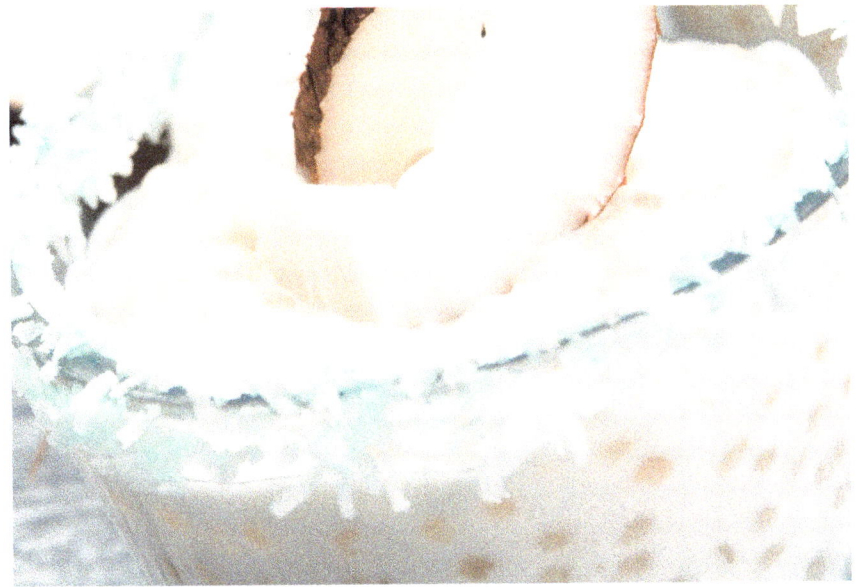

This dessert is soy-free and gluten-free! Enjoy warm or cold.

Use a 3 to 4 quart (3-4 L) slow cooker.

Makes 6 servings.

Ingredients:

- 1 teaspoon (5 ml) vanilla extract
- 2 teaspoons (10 ml) orange extract
- ½ cup (120 ml) small pearl tapioca
- 4 cups (960 ml) coconut milk or almond milk
- Sweetener (maple syrup) is optional

Directions:

Combine all ingredients in the slow cooker and allow to cook on low for 3 ½ to 4 ½ hours, or on high for 2 hours. Add sweetener as desired. After finished, set in the refrigerator for a few hours.

44 - Rice Pudding

For a quick, but tasty dessert, try this rice pudding. 100% vegan and delicious, rice pudding will be sure to please all.

Use a 4 quart (4 L) slow cooker.

Makes 8 servings.

Ingredients:

- Pinch of salt
- ½ teaspoon (2.5 ml) cinnamon
- 1 teaspoon (5 ml) vanilla
- 3 tablespoons (45 ml) vegan margarine
- ¼ cup (60 ml) dried cranberries or cherries (optional)
- ¼ cup (60 ml) chopped dried apricots (optional)
- 1 cup (240 ml) uncooked rice
- 1 cup (240 ml) sugar
- 4 cups (960 ml) vanilla almond milk

Directions:

Add all ingredients to your slow cooker, and allow to cook for 2 to 4 hours on low. Occasionally stir, and serve warm or cold.

45 - Healthy Brownies

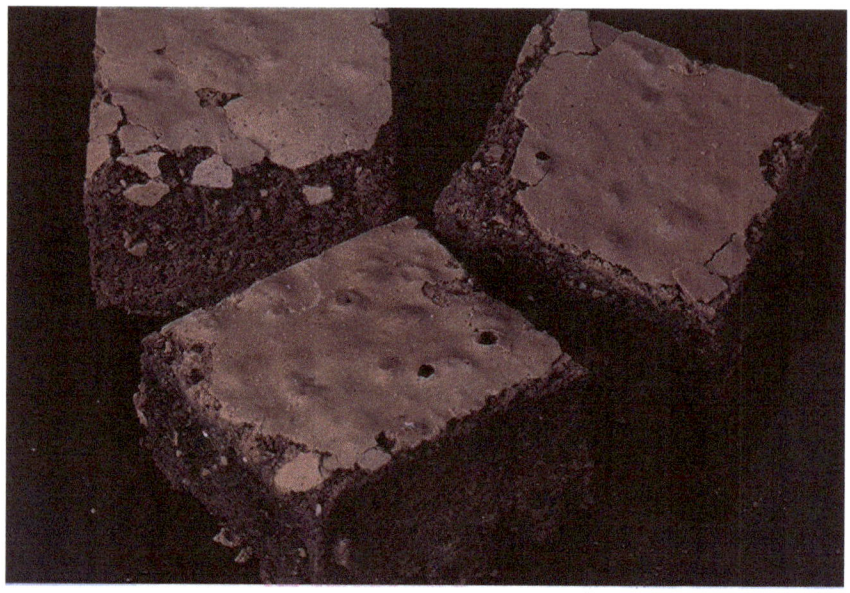

Brownies may seem the complete opposite of vegan food, but now they can be enjoyed as completely animal-free! Serve warm over vegan vanilla ice cream for a special treat.

Use a 2 ½ to 3 quart (2.5-3 L) slow cooker.

Ingredients:

- 1 ½ teaspoons (7.5 ml) baking powder
- 1 tablespoon (15 ml) coconut oil
- 2 tablespoons (30 ml) Ener-G egg replacement
- ½ cup (120 ml) water
- ½ cup (120 ml) unsweetened cocoa powder
- ½ cup (120 ml) walnuts (optional)
- ¾ cup (180 ml) unsweetened apple sauce
- 6 oz (168 g) unsweetened vegan baker's chocolate or 6 squares
- 1 cup (240 ml) maple syrup
- 1 cup (240 ml) whole wheat pastry flour
- 2 mashed medium size, ripe bananas
- Olive oil in oil sprayer

Directions:

Spray the inside of the slow cooker with oil after lining the bottom with parchment. Mix the baking powder, cocoa powder, and flour in a bowl. Melt the vegan chocolate in a microwave for 2 minutes, and then in 30 second intervals while stirring between intervals until melted. Then add the coconut oil to the chocolate and stir. Mix Ener-G egg replacer with ½ cup (120 ml) water. Mix the egg replacer in a bowl with the chocolate, and stir in maple syrup, mashed bananas, and applesauce. Whisk in the flour mixture and mix everything well. Pour it into the slow cooker and allow to cook for 4 hours on low, or until a knife can be pulled out of the brownies and remain clean. Allow the slow cooker to cool and flip upside down to remove.

46 - Apple Cobbler

Make warm, fresh apple cobbler with all vegan ingredients! Enjoy warm in the fall with fresh apples.

Use a 4 quart (4 L) slow cooker.

Makes 6 servings.

Ingredients:

- ¼ teaspoon (1.25 ml) cinnamon
- 2 tablespoons (30 ml) flour
- 3 tablespoons (45 ml) melted vegan margarine
- ⅓ cup (80 ml) sugar
- ⅓ cup (80 ml) dried cranberries
- ⅔ cup (160 ml) rolled oats
- ¾ cup (180 ml) brown sugar
- 1 cup (240 ml) water
- 4 ½ cups (1,080 ml) cored, peeled and sliced apples

Directions:

Stir the apples, flour, and white sugar in a bowl so that the apples are coated. Then add cinnamon, cranberries and oats, continuing to stir all ingredients. Add the mixture and water to the slow cooker. Mix well before drizzling margarine and brown sugar over top. Allow to cook for 4 to 6 hours on low.

47 - Pumpkin Pie Pudding

Feel like you are in the fall with pumpkin pie pudding! Enjoy this recipe instead of actual pumpkin pie for a healthier dessert.

Use a 2 to 3 quart (2-3 L) slow cooker.

Makes 8 servings.

Ingredients:

- 2 teaspoons (10 ml) vanilla
- 2 ½ teaspoons (12.5 ml) pumpkin pie spice
- 3 teaspoons (15 ml) Ener-G egg replacer
- 2 tablespoons (30 ml) melted vegan margarine
- ¼ cup (60 ml) brown sugar
- ¼ cup (60 ml) water
- ½ cup (120 ml) sugar
- ½ cup (120 ml) Bisquick
- 1 ⅓ cups (320 ml) nondairy creamer
- 1 can (15 oz or 420 g) pumpkin

Directions:

Mix dry Ener-G with ¼ cup water (60 ml). Combine mixture in a bowl with all ingredients and mix well. Spray oil in the slow cooker and put mixture in the slow cooker. Allow to cook for 7 to 8 hours on low.

48 - Pumpkin Bread

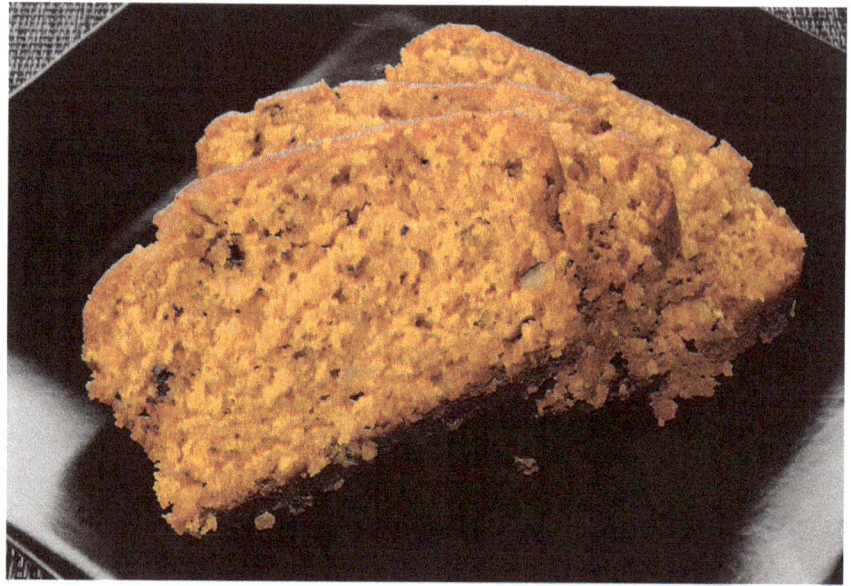

This pumpkin bread recipe will make you crave for more. For a different way of eating, use the same recipe to bake in muffin tins.

Makes 4 to 6 servings

Ingredients:

- ¼ teaspoon (1.25 ml) salt
- ½ teaspoon (2.5 ml) cinnamon
- ½ teaspoon (2.5 ml) nutmeg
- 1 teaspoon (5 ml) baking soda
- 3 teaspoons (15 ml) Ener-G egg replacer
- ¼ cup (60 ml) water
- ½ cup (120 ml) oil
- ½ cup (120 ml) sugar
- ½ cup (120 ml) packed brown sugar
- 1 ½ cup (360 ml) flour
- 15 oz can (420 g) pumpkin

Directions:

Mix the Ener-G egg replacer with ¼ cup (60 ml) water. In a bowl, mix the oil, sugar, and brown sugar. Add the egg replacer and pumpkin while stirring. Lastly, put in the remaining dry ingredients and blend well. Pour the mixture into a bread pan, sprayed with oil to prevent sticking. Pour two cups (480 ml) of water into your slow cooker and carefully set the pan on top. Before covering the slow cooker with the lid, set 8 to 10 paper towels on top to capture the condensation and prevent the bread from getting soggy. Allow to cook for 2 ½ to 3 hours on high.

49 - Banana Brown Betty

For a unique treat, try this tasty recipe. Warm and sweet, it is sure to satisfy your cravings and more.

Use a 4 quart (4 L) slow cooker.

Ingredients:

- ⅛ teaspoon (0.6 ml) salt
- ¼ teaspoon (1.25 ml) ground ginger
- ¼ teaspoon (1.25 ml) ground nutmeg
- ½ teaspoon (2.5 ml) ground cinnamon
- 2 tablespoons (30 ml) brandy or rum
- ¼ cup (60 ml) unsweetened almond milk
- ⅓ cup (80 ml) chopped toasted pecans
- ⅓ cup (80 ml) packed light brown sugar or granulated natural sugar
- ⅓ cup (80 ml) pure maple syrup
- 6 cups (1,440 ml) cubed white bread
- 4 ripe peeled and chopped bananas

Directions:

Mix salt, nutmeg, ginger, cinnamon, almond milk, and maple syrup in a bowl. Then stir in and coat the bread crumbs. Mix brandy, sugar, pecans, and bananas in a separate bowl. Spray the inside of slow cooker with oil. Pour half of the bread mixture into the slow cooker, spread, and then add half of the banana mixture on top. Repeat so that there are four different layers of the alternating mixtures. Allow to cook for 1 ½ to 2 hours on high. Serve while warm.

50 - Vegan Fudge

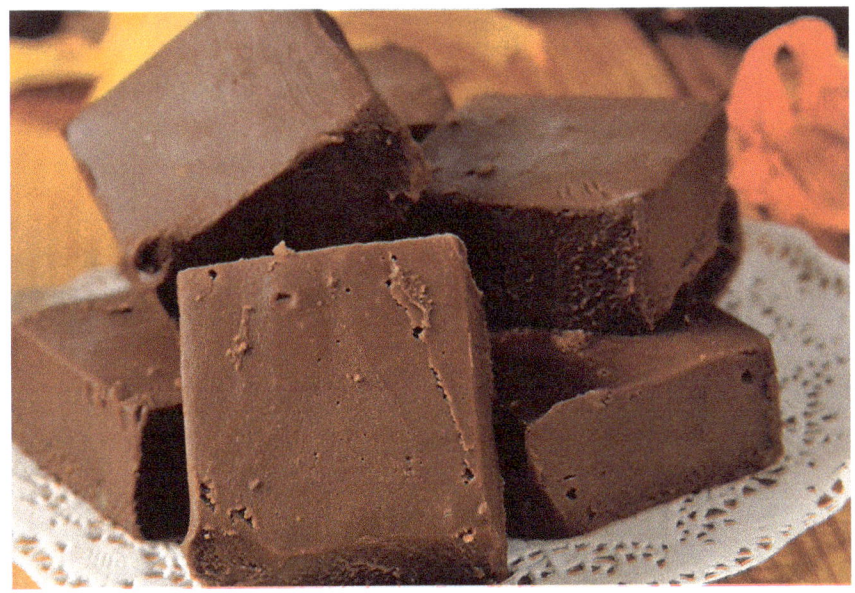

Fudge is usually difficult to make, but this recipe makes it easy! Enjoy as a special treat any time of day.

Use a 2 to 3 quart (2-3 L) slow cooker.

Ingredients:

- Dash of sea salt
- 1 teaspoon (5 ml) vanilla extract
- ¼ cup (60 ml) coconut milk
- ¼ cup (60 ml) maple syrup
- 2 ½ cups (600 g) vegan chocolate chips (Trader Joe's)

Directions:

Combine salt, maple syrup, coconut milk, and chocolate chips in your slow cooker and stir. Allow to cook for 2 hours on low, keeping the lid on. Then after turning the cooker off, add the vanilla and stir to combine. It is important that the fudge is left to cool to room temperature with the cooker lid off, which takes about 4 hours. After 4 hours, stir the fudge with a spoon (may be difficult, but keep stirring until it loosens). This will take 5 to 10 minutes. Use a 1-quart (1 L) casserole dish sprayed with oil (to prevent sticking) and pour the fudge in. Set in the fridge to cool for at least 4 hours.

Thank You

If you enjoyed the meal plan, please consider leaving a review of the book. Good reviews encourage an author to write as well as help books to sell. Good reviews can be just a few short sentences describing what you liked about the book. If you could spend 30 seconds writing a review, I would appreciate it. You can review this title right now at your favorite retailer.

As a perk for purchasing this book, you can get a printable meal plan and shopping list by signing up for my newsletter at the link below:

https://gotorecipecookbooks.com/vegan-sc/

Other Books by Rachel Richards

- The 7-Day Ketogenic Diet Meal Plan: 35 Delicious Low Carb Recipes For Weight Loss Motivation - Volume 1

- The 7-Day Ketogenic Diet Meal Plan: 35 Delicious Low Carb Recipes For Weight Loss Motivation - Volume 2

- The 7-Day Ketogenic Diet Meal Plan: 35 Delicious Low Carb Recipes For Weight Loss Motivation - Volume 3

- The 7-Day Ketogenic Diet Meal Plan: 35 Delicious Low Carb Recipes For Weight Loss Motivation - Volumes 1 to 3

- The 7-Day Gluten Free Diet Plan: 35 Healthy Wheat Free Recipes To Banish Your Wheat Belly – Volume 1

Get the latest update on new releases from the author at:

https://rachelrichardsrecipebooks.com/newsletter/

About the Author – Rachel Richards

Rachel Richards enjoys creating specialized cookbooks for those who are health-conscious.

Visit Rachel's website at:

https://rachelrichardsrecipebooks.com/

Connect with Rachel Richards

I really appreciate you reading my book! Here are my social media contact information:

Friend me on Facebook: https://www.facebook.com/rachelrichardsrecipebooks

Follow me on Twitter: https://twitter.com/rachlrichards

Check me out on Goodreads: https://www.goodreads.com/author/show/14172765.Rachel_Richards

Subscribe to my newsletter: https://rachelrichardsrecipebooks.com/newsletter/

Visit my website: https://rachelrichardsrecipebooks.com/

www.ingramcontent.com/pod-product-compliance
Lightning Source LLC
Chambersburg PA
CBHW061803070526
44586CB00023B/2698